How To Get Rid Of Agonizing Knee Pain

I0417534

17 Agonizing Knee Problems... And The Surefire Solutions To Erase Them!

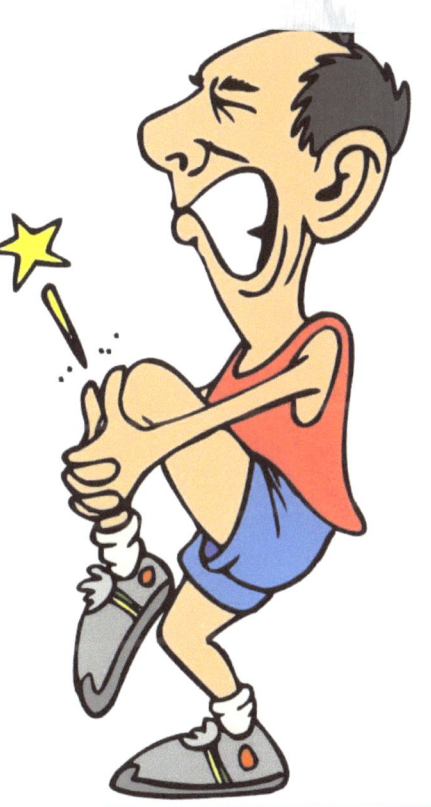

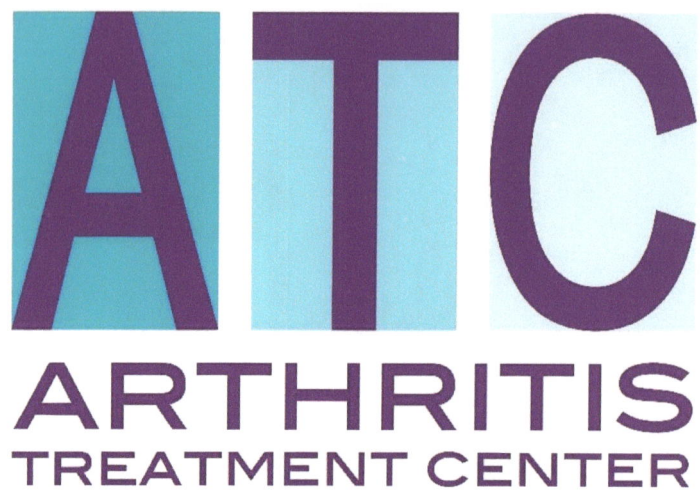

Nathan Wei, MD, FACP, FACR
Arthritis Treatment Center
71 Thomas Johnson Drive
Frederick, MD 21702

Contents

Preface 5

Chapter 1 11

Structure and function 11

Chapter Two..14

Bursitis...14

Chapter Three..17

Tendinitis..17

Chapter Four 22

Medial plica syndrome 22

Chapter Five...23

Pellegrini Stieda disease 23

Chapter 6 24

Nerve related knee pain 24

Chapter 7 27

Patellofemoral pain syndrome............................27

Chapter 8 29

Bakers cyst 29

Chapter 9 31

Chapter 10...33

Mechanical knee pain 33

Chapter 11 35

Chapter 12...37

Arthritis..37

Conclusion:...46

About the Author...48

Preface

Knee pain is often due to arthritis and related conditions which is why I'm writing this book. To provide some insight into the types of conditions that can cause knee pain, who to see, when to see them, what types of problems can cause knee pain, and how to diagnose and manage it. I'm also providing tips on newer therapies that might be appropriate for you. Often patients aren't privy to more advanced techniques and end up having painful, expensive, and often ineffective surgery.

I'd like to make sure that doesn't happen to you.

First though, I want to provide you some insight into why I'm so passionate about arthritis treatment. I'm going to be revealing things about myself that are somewhat painful but I think important.

I'm probably a lot like you. I'm preparing this book in June 2016 and I was born in August 1949 so my 67th birthday is coming up soon. If the surveys we've conducted on our website are any indication I'm smack dab in the middle age range of those people who seem to be most interested in arthritis. We're Baby Boomers and now the health problems of Baby Boomers, especially arthritis, are of increasing concern because we all want to stay active and healthy.

Another reason I think I have something in common with many of you is that I have arthritis. I have osteoarthritis in my neck, both ankles, and right hip. The results of athletic injuries when I was younger. So I deal with aches and pains too.

My first encounter with arthritis was in college when I went out to California to visit some relatives. One of the relatives I visited was a great aunt who had horrible rheumatoid arthritis. She was confined to a wheelchair and was literally frozen in place. At that time in the 1960's there wasn't a whole lot that could be done and she died about a year later from the complications of her disease and the complications of the high doses of cortisone she got for her arthritis.

Ironically enough, 18 years ago I encountered rheumatoid arthritis again. It was Thanksgiving and our family was together. My sister Esther asked me to look at her feet. They had been bothering her for several months. She had seen a

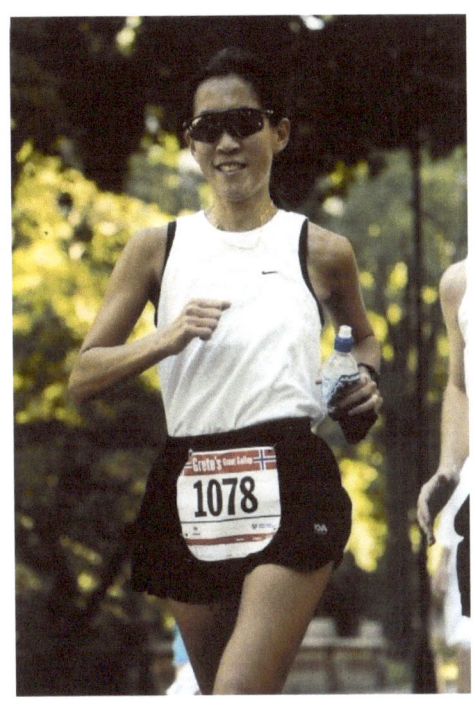

A Photo of my sister, Esther

podiatrist and an orthopedic surgeon. I took one look and my heart sank. I looked at her wrists and hands. Esther had rheumatoid arthritis. I put her in touch with a rheumatology colleague of mine in New York City where she lived. And fortunately... after a rocky start, Esther got on the right medicines and improved dramatically. So much so that she took a new hobby.... running. She started running marathons.

But arthritis didn't leave my family alone. Let me tell you about my son, Benji.

My son, Benji, was playing travel soccer and at the age of 10, developed severe knee pain.

Initially my wife and I thought it was a sports injury.

It got worse and we took him to see numerous doctors.... orthopedic surgeons... who told us they though it was an arthritis problem... pediatric rheumatologists diagnosed various other things.

My wife and I didn't know what was happening. We felt powerless. Benji was getting worse daily. There were some days when I literally had to carry him in my arms from his bed downstairs to the kitchen so he could eat breakfast before going to school. You have to remember that a doctor with a sick child is a parent first. Even though I am an adult rheumatologist, pediatric rheumatology is a completely different animal. I was so frustrated.

Out of desperation, I remembered one of my medical school classmates, Dr. Tom Lehman, was a pediatric rheumatologist at the Hospital for Special Surgery in New York. So I called him and asked, "Tom, would you do me a favor and see my son Benji?" Tom said, "It would be an honor…" So my wife, Judy, took Benji to see Dr. Lehman.

He took one look at Benji and knew right away what the problem was. Juvenile ankylosing spondylitis, and also recognized how badly Benji was doing. He started Benji out on disease modifying medicines and biologics and soon Benji went into remission.

Benji went on to play soccer in high school and then rugby in college. He graduated from Bowdoin College in 2013.

So… there you have it. This is why I view arthritis as something to conquer and I'm on a crusade of sorts. For my patients…. For my family.

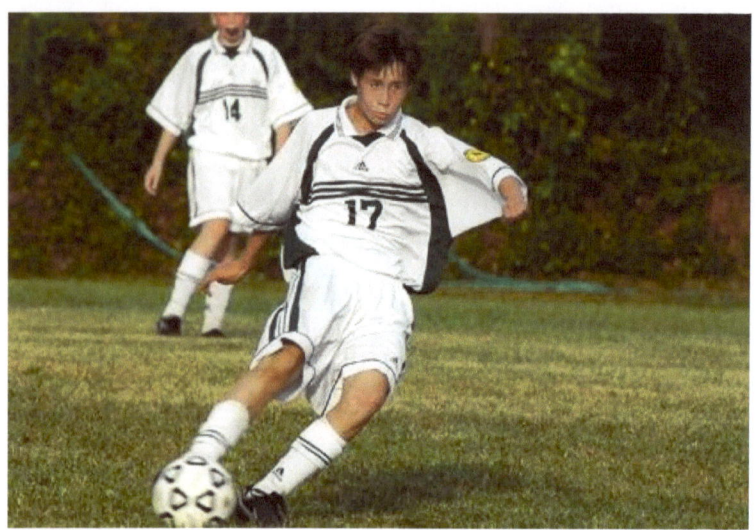

Benji playing soccer.

Chapter 1
Structure and function

The knee joint is complicated. It consists of four bones, the upper leg bone, the femur, and two lower leg bones, the tibia and fibula, and finally the patella or kneecap.

The knee is held together by a

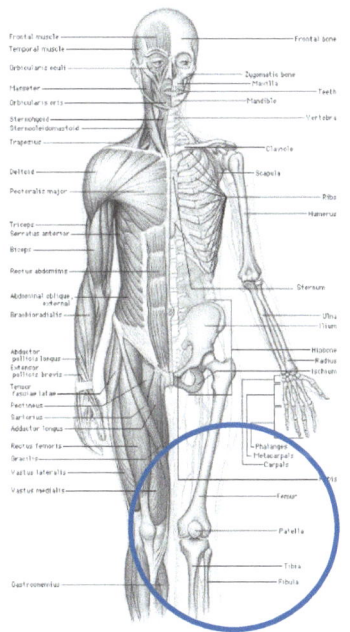

structured arrangement of ligaments. These are the medial collateral ligament along the inside of the knee, lateral collateral ligament along the outside part of the knee, and the anterior and posterior cruciate

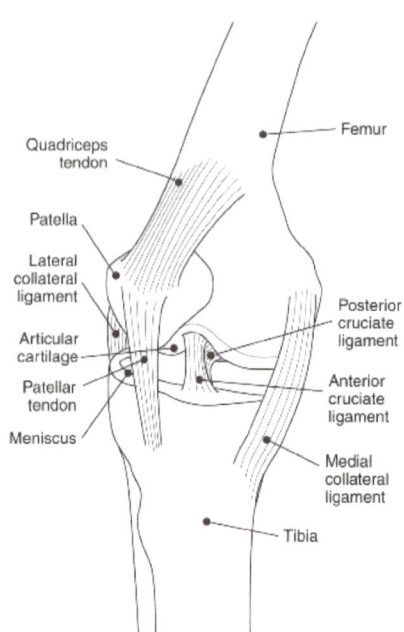

ligaments located within the knee. The latter two ligaments prevent excessive forward and backward motion of the knee joint. In addition, the knee is surrounded by a complex arrangement of tendons, muscles, and bursae. Bursae are small fluid-filled sacs that act as shock absorbers around the knee.

The knee structure inside is also complicated. The ends of the long bones, specifically the femur and tibia, are covered by a thin layer of extremely tough hyaline cartilage. Hyaline cartilage is designed to contend with both impact loading as well as shear forces.

In addition to the hyaline cartilage, there are two pieces of fibrocartilage. These are called the menisci. There is both medial meniscus as well as a lateral meniscus. These help to further cushion the knee and allow the knee to move in different directions.

The entire knee joint is enclosed in an envelope lined with a tissue called synovium. Synovial cells produce a small amount of joint fluid that helps both lubricate as well as nourish cartilage. As mentioned earlier, the two cruciate ligaments, anterior and posterior, prevent excessive forward and backward movement of the knee joint.

The major functions of the knee are to bear weight and to absorb shock. The knee accomplishes this through a variety of motions. First and foremost, the knee is a hinge joint. However, there is also a rotational component as well as a gliding component. All three of these motions are critical to normal functioning of the knee joint.

Chapter Two
Bursitis

Bursae are small sacs of fluid that cushion joints. They're located throughout the body. There are an abundant number of bursae that surround and protect the knee. These bursae are located above, in front of, and below the knee. When they become inflamed, they can become swollen and painful.

Bursitis symptoms include swelling, heat, redness, and pain. In severe circumstances, patients can also develop fever and chills.

Anserine bursitis is common in middle-aged, elderly, and overweight individuals. The pain of anserine bursitis is located two inches below and along the medial part of the knee. The pain is aggravated by walking as well as negotiating stairs. Anserine bursitis is often a complication of osteoarthritis of the knee. Because of this, it is often overlooked.

The treatment of anserine bursitis includes rest as well as stretching of the tendons that form the anserine bursa (semitendinosus, gracilis, and semimembranosus).

Glucocorticoid injections can also be effective. While anserine bursitis usually gets better with this treatment approach, it has a tendency to recur particularly in overweight individuals.

Prepatellar bursitis is bursitis that is located in front of the patella or kneecap. It is usually due to trauma – in particular, frequent kneeling. The key thing about prepatellar bursitis is to make sure that the bursa is not infected. Aspiration of fluid from the prepatellar bursa using ultrasound guidance is recommended. Any fluid that is obtained should be sent for culture. Patients with an infected bursa need to be started on antibiotic therapy.

Infrapatellar bursitis refers to bursitis involving a bursa located just below the patella. This type of bursitis is almost always due to trauma. However it can be seen in other conditions such as rheumatoid arthritis.

The treatment for both prepatellar and infrapatellar bursitis is identical. The first rule is to make sure that there is no infection. Protecting the knee using knee pads is often helpful. Patients may require a short course of nonsteroidal anti-inflammatory drugs or NSAIDs. Ice and rest are also helpful.

Chapter Three
Tendinitis

Tendons are pieces of tissue and ropes that connect muscles or bones. Over time, tendons can become irritated and worn by repetitive stress. Tendon afflictions are a frequent cause of knee pain.

The quadriceps tendon connects the thigh muscles to the patella. Tendon damage here can often lead to catastrophic consequences such as tendon rupture. Risk factors for quadriceps tendon rupture include kidney disease, steroid therapy, rheumatoid arthritis, gout, and the use of fluoroquinolone antibiotics. In fact, the FDA, in 2016 issued what is called a black box warning in regards to the use of fluoroquinolone antibiotics because of this very issue.

Quadriceps tendon abnormalities are uncommon. They are usually caused by trauma or other stressors.

When quadriceps tendon rupture does occur, it is characterized by severe pain as well as inability to straighten the leg. Surgery is required. The recovery period, as one might imagine, is long.

The patellar tendon connects the patella to the tibia or shinbone. Patellar tendinitis is common in athletes who engage in running, jumping, and kicking. Therefore runners, basketball players, tennis players, and soccer players are those who are at greatest risk. Patellar tendinitis is often referred to as "jumpers knee."

Symptoms include pain, tenderness of the tendon, and inability to straighten the leg. If not attended to properly, the patellar tendon can rupture. If this occurs, surgery is required.

The treatment for both quadriceps and patellar tendinitis include rest, racing, ice, nonsteroidal anti-inflammatory drugs, and stretching. However, the treatment of choice in order to both relieve pain as well as restore function is the use of ultrasound-guided platelet rich plasma (PRP) injection.

Platelet rich plasma is an ultra-concentrate of blood. This ultra-concentrate is obtained by centrifugation of a patient's blood in order to obtain platelets. Platelets are cells that are rich in growth and healing factors. Using local anesthetic, the damaged and/or diseased tendon is peppered with small holes using a small gauge needle in order to induce injury. Injury is the first step in healing. This peppering is done using ultrasound guidance. The PRP is then injected into the treated area.

Hamstring tendons connect the pelvis to the back of the knee. The hamstrings help with walking as well as with running.

Hamstring tendinitis generally occurs in athletes who are involved in running and jumping. The pain is felt either in the buttock region at the origin or behind the knee at the insertion.

High hamstring tendonitis causes pain in the "sitbone" with sitting and walking. Low hamstring tendonitis is felt in the back of the knee and sometimes the calf. The pain of hamstring tendinitis is aggravated by weight-bearing. The diagnosis is suspected by clinical examination and confirmed by magnetic resonance imaging or MRI.

Diagnostic ultrasound is also an excellent method for visualizing hamstring injury. Hamstring tendinitis is treated using rest, ice, physical therapy, nonsteroidal anti-inflammatory drugs, and platelet rich plasma administered using ultrasound guidance.

The popliteus tendon is also located in the back of the knee laterally. Popliteus tendinitis is often associated with hamstring tendinitis. The pain is located at the outside back of the knee and is aggravated by downhill running. On examination there is tenderness and pain. The diagnosis is suspected by clinical examination and confirmed by magnetic resonance imaging or diagnostic ultrasound.

As with the other forms of tendinitis mentioned earlier, the treatment involves rest, ice, physical therapy, nonsteroidal anti-inflammatory drugs, and platelet rich plasma injection.

Chapter Four
Medial plica syndrome

The medial plica is a fold of synovium or joint lining tissue located inside the medial part of the knee. When this fold of synovium becomes trapped between the patella and the upper leg bone, there can be pain, snapping, and clicking along the medial aspect of the knee.

When viewed arthroscopically, the plica appears thickened and inflamed.

The medial plica syndrome is treated using arthroscopy with removal of the plica.

Chapter Five
Pellegrini Stieda disease

Pellegrini-Stieda disease refers to a condition where the medial collateral ligament becomes calcified. Pain is located on the inside (medial) part of the knee. There is reduced range of motion. The diagnosis is often made by x-ray where a small area of calcification is seen involving the medial collateral ligament. Fortunately this problem usually gets better spontaneously.

It is rare that any further intervention is required.

Chapter 6
Nerve related knee pain

Three major nerves surround the knee. Two of them can be associated with significant knee pain. The pain coming from nerves is usually due to pressure or trauma involving the nerves. The key take away message here is that nerve-related pain can be mistaken for other problems.

The sciatic nerve originates from nerve roots in the low back. When irritated sciatic nerve pain is felt behind and on the outside part of the knee. The tragic thing about this is that some people have actually had knee surgery when the problem was actually coming from the back.

The peroneal nerve is located on the outside part of the knee. It can be damaged by trauma or by stretching. For example, women who are having extensive gynecologic surgery with her feet in stirrups often times can develop peroneal nerve trauma. Until recently, one cause of peroneal nerve injury was the use of knee replacement hardware that was not custom fit to the patient. Often, women would receive knee replacement parts met for men. The edges of these replacements would rub on the peroneal nerve causing post-operative pain.

Peroneal nerve injury symptoms included pain as well as numbness and tingling on the outside of the leg below the knee extending into the foot. When severe, foot drop would occur. Fortunately, this type of problem is not that frequent.

The diagnosis is suspected by history and physical examination, confirmed by electrical studies as well as by MRI.

The treatment involves removing whatever is pressing on the nerve. Occasionally, ultrasound-guided hydro-dissection can help relieve the nerve pain. Hydro-dissection involves injecting a large volume of fluid in the sheath located just outside the nerve, thereby relieving pressure on the nerve. In cases where conservative management is not effective, neurosurgical consultation is required.

Chapter 7
Patellofemoral pain syndrome

Patellofemoral pain syndrome refers to pain as well as a sensation of crunching that occurs between the patella and the upper leg bone. From the AAOS (American Academy of Orthopaedic Surgeons) "...nerves sense pain in the soft tissues and bone around the kneecap. These soft tissues include the tendons, the fat pad beneath the patella, and the synovial tissue that lines the knee joint.

In some cases of knee pain, a condition called *chondromalacia patella* is present. Chondromalacia patella is the softening and breakdown of the articular cartilage on the underside of the kneecap. There are no nerves in articular cartilage—so damage to the cartilage itself cannot directly cause pain. It can, however, lead to inflammation of the synovium and pain in the underlying bone."

The problem develops usually as a result of either overuse or malalignment of the patella.

Stiffness occurs with sitting. Pain is aggravated with bending as well as with loading the knee, climbing the stairs, and squatting. Patellofemoral pain syndrome is common in younger patients, particularly females.

The treatment of patellofemoral pain syndrome consists of rest, physical therapy, nonsteroidal anti-inflammatory medications, ice, and exercises. Occasionally surgery is required.

Chapter 8
Bakers cyst

A Bakers cyst is a result of buildup of fluid in the back of the knee. It develops as a result of an opening at the back of the knee formed by the confluence of the semimembranosus muscle and the gastrocnemius muscle. Fluid can flow back out of the knee joint through this opening but cannot return. In essence, this is a one way valve.

A Bakers cyst is a common occurrence with different types of arthritis.

Symptoms include pain, stiffness, swelling, and tightness behind the knee.

One complication is that a Baker's cyst can push down into the calf and rupture. It then looks like a blood clot. It is mandatory that a venous Doppler study be performed in order to exclude the presence of a true blood clot.

The diagnosis of a Baker's cyst can be suspected clinically and confirmed by diagnostic ultrasound or MRI. Again, it is important to rule out an associated blood clot.

The treatment of a Baker's cyst can involve removal of fluid from the Baker's cyst with injection of glucocorticoid. This is very effective for symptomatic relief although the Baker's cyst can return. If the Baker's cyst recurs often, surgery may be required.

Chapter 9

Synovitis refers to swelling of the lining of the joint. Synovial cells can be irritated by any number of different stimuli. When this occurs, inflammatory cells migrate to the area and inflammation involving the synovial cells is magnified. This is referred to as synovitis. Synovitis is common with many different types of arthritis.

Synovitis can cause swelling of the knee joint. Also, if the synovial cells produce an excessive amount of fluid in response to inflammation, fluid accumulation can occur inside the knee joint. This is found with most inflammatory disorders such as rheumatoid arthritis, psoriatic arthritis, Reiter's disease, gout, pseudogout, and even osteoarthritis.

To follow up on that, the fluid accumulation that occurs inside the knee is referred to as an effusion. Sometimes it is called "water on the knee." Knee effusions can occur not only as a result of trauma and arthritis, but also with certain metabolic abnormalities such as hemophilia.

Chapter 10
Mechanical knee pain

Mechanical knee pain refers to structural damage occurring inside the knee. An example might be tearing of the menisci, the fibrocartilage cushions inside the knee. Damage to the

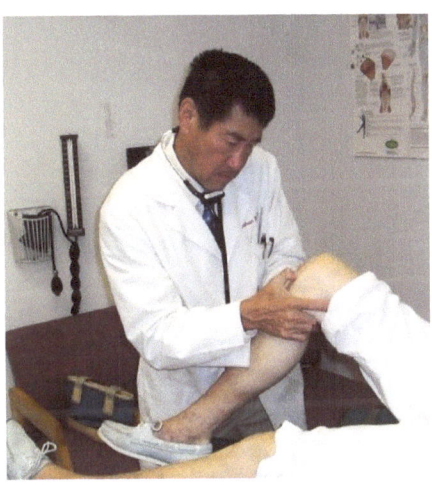

Nathan Wei, MD examining a patient with knee pain.

stronger hyaline cartilage covering of the bones inside the knee may also cause mechanical dysfunction. Tearing of ligaments, particularly the cruciate ligaments can cause mechanical knee pain.

The diagnosis is suspected clinically and may be confirmed by imaging studies such as MRI. The treatment for mechanical disorders may be medical or surgical depending on a number of different factors including the severity of the disorder, effect on activity, and amount of pain.

Chapter 11

Osteochondritis dissecans is a condition where bone beneath the cartilage of a joint dies due to lack of blood flow. This section of bone and cartilage can then break loose, causing pain and limitation of joint motion.

Why this occurs is generally unknown although trauma can certainly play a role. Osteochondritis dissecans can cause severe pain. The treatment involves an arthroscopic procedure where the loose piece of bone and cartilage is removed and a new piece of cartilage is plugged into the defect. Non-weight bearing for several months after the procedure is required.

Chapter 12
Arthritis

Many types of arthritis affect the knee. These include rheumatoid arthritis, osteoarthritis, gout, pseudogout, urethritis of psoriasis, Reiter's disease, Lyme disease, and septic processes.

The diagnosis of arthritis is made using clinical observation and examination, laboratory testing, evaluation of joint fluid if available, and diagnostic imaging.

The treatment of arthritis depends on the underlying type of arthritis involved.

Of special interest is osteoarthritis. This is the most common type of arthritis and probably affects more than 40,000,000

Americans. This is a disease of articular cartilage, the hyaline cartilage that caps the ends of long bones. While it used to be thought that osteoarthritis was primarily a "wear and tear" disease, we now know that the development of osteoarthritis is extremely complicated and involves a convoluted interaction of cartilage, bone, synovium, and many other factors.

Osteoarthritis is a baby boomer affliction and the incidence is expected to explode in the next few years. Approximately 25 years ago, the Center for Disease Control (CDC) in Atlanta stated in their newsletter that "100,000 Americans cannot get from the bed to the bathroom because of osteoarthritis affecting the hip or knee". Obviously, that number has risen dramatically.

Unfortunately, the treatment of osteoarthritis, until recently, has been aimed at symptomatic relief only. Modalities that have been used include ice, various exercises, physical therapy, bracing, nonsteroidal anti-inflammatory medications, analgesics, and injections of glucocorticoids or lubricants.

One of the major considerations is weight loss. The mechanical advantages of weight loss are obvious. Less weight means less stress on the joints. However, there is also a biologic reason. Fat cells contain leptins which are proteins that promote inflammation. Obviously, the more fat cells the patient has, the more inflammation there will be.

While many of these pain-relieving treatments may be effective, they also carry with them the potential for side effects. In particular, nonsteroidal anti-inflammatory drugs have been associated not only with gastrointestinal complications such as bleeding ulcers but also with a marked increased incidence of cardiovascular events such as heart attack and stroke.

Also, some of the treatments from the past that have been felt to be effective have recently found to be totally ineffective. An example would be acetaminophen. This used to be listed as a first line therapy for osteoarthritis in many therapeutic recommendations, among them being the American College of Rheumatology guidelines. However, recent data has shown that acetaminophen is ineffective for relieving the pain associated with osteoarthritis of the knee. There have been more recent breakthroughs in the quest for improved symptomatic relief for osteoarthritis.

These include injectable types of therapies such as direct injections into the joint with capsaicin, the active compound in hot chili peppers, as well as purified serum human albumin. The latter has been shown to have mild to moderate disease modifying effects as well.

Antibodies to nerve growth factor have been studied extensively. This therapy relies on the ability to block pain signals and is extremely effective for relieving the pain of osteoarthritis. Clinical trials are ongoing.

Resurgent interest in the use of complementary therapies such as acupuncture, medicinal herbs, and other natural anti-inflammatory compounds has occurred.

Acupuncture has been found in multiple clinical trials to be effective for pain relief for osteoarthritis.

Herbal therapies such as curcumin, Boswellia, bromelain, fish oil, glucosamine, chondroitin, ginger, garlic, and others have also been found to be helpful.

Of special interest has been the development of regenerative therapies for osteoarthritis. Multiple biologic growth factors have been studied and the ability to heal damage to cartilage and regrow cartilage has been exciting news for clinicians.

A number of growth factors are undergoing clinical trial as possible candidates for regeneration of cartilage in osteoarthritis.

Platelet-rich plasma (PRP), an ultra-concentrate of blood also has been demonstrated to have cartilage regenerative effects. Platelet-rich plasma is obtained from a patient's blood sample. This blood specimen is then processed using a special centrifuge in order to obtain a small volume of fluid containing a high concentration of platelets. Platelets are cells that are packed with growth and healing factors. Using ultrasound or arthroscopic guidance, platelet-rich plasma can be administered into an area of injury and there are reports indicating significant cartilage growth occurs.

A tremendous amount of interest has been demonstrated in the potential of various stem cells to help regrow cartilage. Stem cells are blank slate cells located in a variety of tissues such as a bone marrow, fat,

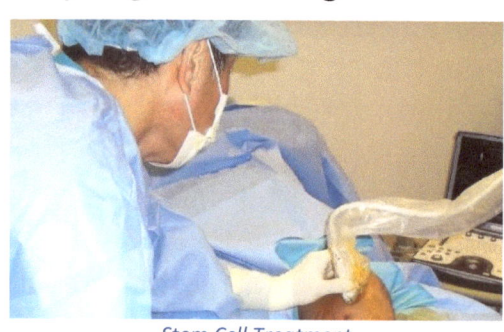

Stem Cell Treatment
Arthritis Treatment Center

periosteum of bone, and even peripheral blood. Among the various types of stem cells that have been studied include embryonic stem cells, allogeneic or donor stem cells, autologous stem cells—a person's own stem cells, and a new type of stem cell called the-induced pluri-potential stem cell.

Obviously, these types of therapies are still considered investigational but look extremely promising.

A practical approach to the management of osteoarthritis shows that there is a dichotomy between medical practitioners such as rheumatologists and orthopedic surgeons. It is the job of the rheumatologist to try to keep the patient from having to have surgery if possible.

Arthroscopic debridement of an osteoarthritic joint may be helpful. There have been conflicting studies regarding the efficacy of debridement for the osteoarthritic knee. However, in certain cases where an inflammatory component is prominent, arthroscopy—meaning the use of a small telescope designed to look inside the joint—may be found to be helpful in removing damage and disease tissue. This certainly makes sense if regenerative therapies are considered as the second stage of treatment.

Recently, a tiny arthroscope, the size of a 14 gauge needle has been designed to help with imaging. We have found it very useful, particularly when imaging procedures such as MRI are either contraindicated or too expensive.

In those patients where surgical treatment is the only option, with two types of surgeries that are available are cartilage sparing and cartilage sacrificing.

The cartilage sparing type of surgical procedure is called an osteotomy. This involves the removal of a wedge of bone from the patient's tibia in order to help straighten out the angulation abnormality. This is often used in young patients to help buy time until the joint can be replaced.

Cartilage sacrificing types of treatments include either partial joint replacement or total joint replacement. Progress in the use of total joint replacement has been impressive and is certainly more effective than it was even ten years ago. One of the major issues though is the explosion in the number of joint replacement surgeries occurring at the present time. It is doubtful whether the current healthcare system can sustain this rate of growth.

Conclusion:

There are many conditions that cause knee pain. An accurate diagnosis and a well thought out treatment plan can provide relief.

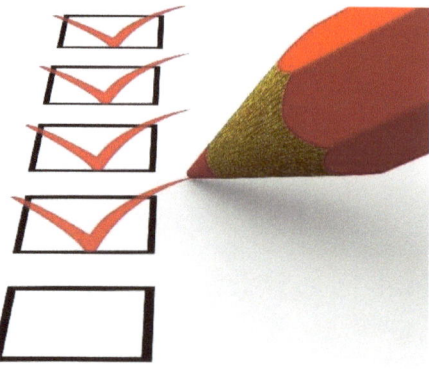

New advances in regenerative medicine look very promising.

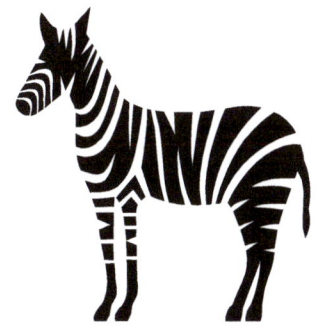
This book should not be a substitute for a thorough examination by your physician. The products that are mentioned in this book are recommended. Prior to using any of them, we recommend you seek advice from a qualified specialist. Neither the publisher nor the author may be held liable for any injury, loss, or damage sustained by anyone who relies on the information contained in the book.

About the Author

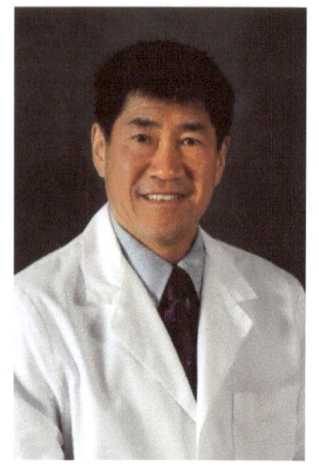

Nathan Wei, MD is a graduate of Swarthmore College and the Jefferson Medical College. He completed his residency at the University of Michigan Medical Center in Ann Arbor, Michigan and his fellowship in arthritis at the National Institutes of Health in Bethesda, Maryland. Dr. Wei is an acknowledged national expert in rheumatoid arthritis and osteoarthritis and is the author of more than 500 publications.

He is a Fellow of the American College of Physicians, a Fellow of the American College of Rheumatology, and is the only American rheumatologist member in the Arthroscopy Association of North America. He is also a member of the American College of Sports Medicine.

Dr. Wei is considered an authority and expert in stem cell and platelet-rich plasma (PRP) procedures, and other innovative techniques. He is active in clinical research and is the Director of the Arthritis Treatment Center, located in Frederick, Maryland.

www.ingramcontent.com/pod-product-compliance
Lightning Source LLC
Chambersburg PA
CBHW050834290526
45792CB00001B/391